COMPLETE GUIDE TO DYSPEPSIA

A Comprehensive Manual For Understanding, Managing, Overcoming Digestive Discomforts With Proven Strategies And Natural Remedies

DEHART HAIRSTON

© [DEHART HAIRSTON], [2024]

All rights reserved. No part of this publication may be reproduced, distributed, or transmitted in any form or by any means, including photocopying, recording, or other electronic or mechanical methods, without the prior written permission of the publisher, except in the case of brief quotations embodied in critical reviews and certain other noncommercial uses permitted by copyright law.

DISCLAIMER

This book's content is only intended for general informative purposes. At the time of writing, the author has taken every precaution to guarantee that the material is correct and current. Nevertheless, the author disclaims all explicit and implicit representations and guarantees about the availability, appropriateness, correctness, completeness, and usefulness of the material on these pages.

Since the author is not a licensed medical practitioner, the material in this book shouldn't be interpreted as medical advice. Before making any modifications to their diet, exercise regimen, or medical treatment, readers are urged to speak with a licensed healthcare provider.

Moreover, the author has no connection to any of the businesses, organizations, or people that are discussed in this book. Any mentions of goods, services, businesses, or people are purely informative and do not indicate endorsement or suggestion.

This book's content is entirely dependent on the author's expertise, study, and comprehension of the topic. Despite having taken reasonable care to offer correct information, the author disclaims all liability for any mistakes or omissions in the material as well as for any losses, harm, or damages resulting from using the information.

It is recommended that readers use their own judgment and discretion when applying the knowledge in this book to their own situations. The use or implementation of any material in this book may result in unfavorable repercussions, directly or indirectly, for which the author assumes no liability.

By reading this book, you agree to release and hold the author harmless from any claims, losses, liabilities, costs, or expenditures resulting from or related to the use of the information you get from it.

Table of Contents

CHAPTER 1 15
- Understanding Dyspepsia 15
- What Is Dyspepsia? 15
- Symptoms And Signs 16
- Common Causes Of Dyspepsia 17
  - 1. Dietary Factors: 17
  - 4. Medications: 18
  - 5. Psychological Factors: 18

CHAPTER 2 21
- Digestive System Basics 21
- Overview Of The Digestive System 21
- How Digestion Works 23
- Role Of Digestive Enzymes And Hormones 24

CHAPTER 3 27
- Lifestyle Factors And Diet 27
- Importance Of Diet In Digestive Health 27
- Foods To Avoid And Foods To Embrace 28
  - 2. Fatty meals: 28
  - 3. Acidic meals: 29
  - 2. Lean Proteins: 29

    3. Probiotic-Rich Foods: 30

    4. Low-Acid Options: 30

  Healthy Eating Habits For Managing Dyspepsia...31

    1. Eat Smaller, More Regular Meals: 31

    2. Chew Food Thoroughly: 31

    3. Avoid Eating Before Bed: 31

    4. Stay Hydrated: 32

    5. Manage Stress: 32

CHAPTER 4 33

  Stress And Its Impact..33

  Relationship Between Stress And Digestive Health 33

  Stress Management Techniques............................34

  Mindfulness And Relaxation Exercises 36

CHAPTER 5 39

  Medications And Dyspepsia 39

  Common Medications That Can Cause Dyspepsia 39

  How To Minimize Medication-Related Symptoms 40

  Consulting Your Doctor About Medication 42

CHAPTER 6 45

  Natural Remedies And Supplements......................45

Herbal Remedies For Dyspepsia 45
Probiotics And Digestive Health 47
Integrating Supplements Safely 48
    1. Consult with a healthcare professional: 48
    2. Investigate possible interactions: 49
    4. Monitor for adverse effects: 49
    5. Give it time: 49

CHAPTER 7 51
Diagnosing Dyspepsia 51
Medical Tests For Identifying Dyspepsia 51
Consulting With Healthcare Professionals 53
    Main Care Physician: 53
    Nutritionist or Dietitian: 54
    Psychologist or Psychiatrist: 54
Understanding Diagnostic Procedures 55
    Process Explanation: 55
    Informed Consent: 55
    Patient Preparation: 56
    During the Procedure: 56
    Post-Procedure Care: 56

CHAPTER 8 59

Treatment Options 59

Lifestyle Changes For Managing Dyspepsia 59

Medical Treatments And Procedures 62

    Antacids: 62

    Proton Pump Inhibitors (PPIs): 62

    Prokinetic Agents: 63

    Antibiotics: 63

    Endoscopic Procedures: 63

    Surgery: 64

Developing A Personalized Treatment Plan 64

    Collaborative Decision-Making: 65

    Regular Follow-Up: 65

    Patient Education: 66

    Multidisciplinary Approach: 66

CHAPTER 9 67

Preventing Dyspepsia 67

Strategies For Preventing Recurrence 67

Long-Term Management Techniques 69

Incorporating Healthy Habits Into Daily Life 72

CHAPTER 10 75

Living Well With Dyspepsia 75

Coping Strategies For Daily Life 75
Support Networks And Resources 77
Thriving Despite Digestive Challenges 78
   CONCLUSION 81
THE END 84

ABOUT THIS BOOK

"Dyspepsia" is more than just a book; it's a thorough guide to understanding, managing, and eventually living despite stomach issues. In today's fast-paced world, when stress, bad food, and pharmaceuticals often wreak havoc on our digestive systems, this book will be an invaluable resource for anybody looking for treatment for dyspepsia and associated conditions.

"Dyspepsia" dives into the fundamental components of this ailment, beginning with a detailed examination of what dyspepsia is and its typical symptoms and causes. It then moves on to give a basic grasp of the digestive tract, informing readers about how digestion works and the roles of numerous enzymes and hormones in the process.

One of this book's most notable elements is its focus on lifestyle and nutrition. Chapter 3 provides useful insights into the role of nutrition in digestive health, advising readers on which foods to avoid and which to embrace, as well as supporting good eating habits that are essential for treating dyspepsia.

Furthermore, "Dyspepsia" goes beyond dietary guidance and discusses the tremendous influence of stress on digestive health in Chapter 4. Providing stress management strategies and mindfulness exercises enables readers to confront stress straight on, reducing its negative effects on their digestive systems.

In Chapter 5, the book delves further into the complex interaction between drugs and dyspepsia, offering practical recommendations for reducing medication-related symptoms and advocating for open communication with healthcare professionals.

Furthermore, "Dyspepsia" recognizes the value of natural therapies and supplements in addressing this ailment. Chapter 6 looks at herbal therapies, probiotics, and safe supplement integration, providing readers with a comprehensive approach to digestive health.

This book provides readers with the information and resources they need to take control of their digestive health, including chapters on diagnosing dyspepsia, treatment choices, and preventative techniques. It highlights the necessity of interacting with healthcare specialists and creating unique treatment regimens based on individual requirements.

Finally, "Dyspepsia" goes beyond basic treatment, empowering readers to live well despite their disease. Chapter 10 offers coping skills for everyday life, supports the formation of support networks, and motivates readers to succeed despite digestive issues.

In summary, "Dyspepsia" is more than just another book on digestive health; it's a lifeline for individuals suffering from dyspepsia, providing hope, advice, and practical answers for regaining control of their health.

CHAPTER 1

Understanding Dyspepsia

What Is Dyspepsia?

Dyspepsia, often known as indigestion, is a frequent word used to describe discomfort or pain in the upper abdomen. It includes a wide spectrum of symptoms that might vary in intensity and duration, making it difficult to identify a single cause. Symptoms of dyspepsia may include bloating, nausea, burping, and a sense of fullness after eating, among others. It is critical to understand that dyspepsia is a symptom of an underlying digestive system issue, not a disease in and of itself.

Understanding dyspepsia requires appreciating its diverse character. While it might be caused by benign factors like overeating or ingesting specific foods, it can also suggest more severe illnesses including gastroesophageal reflux disease (GERD), peptic ulcers, or gastritis. As a result, a thorough knowledge of dyspepsia requires not just recognizing its symptoms, but also identifying probable triggers and underlying problems that contribute to its genesis.

Symptoms And Signs

Recognizing dyspepsia symptoms and indicators is critical for early diagnosis and successful treatment. Dyspepsia patients may report a variety of symptoms, including a burning sensation in the upper belly, bloating, frequent burping, or feeling uncomfortably full even after eating small quantities of food. These symptoms might appear sporadically or repeatedly, often causing pain and a worse quality of life.

Furthermore, dyspepsia symptoms might mimic those of other gastrointestinal problems, making diagnosis difficult without a complete assessment by a healthcare practitioner. It is critical to pay attention to concomitant symptoms such as vomiting, unexpected weight loss, or trouble swallowing, since these may suggest more serious underlying issues that need medical intervention.

Common Causes Of Dyspepsia

Understanding the common causes of dyspepsia is critical for developing effective treatment and preventative methods. Dyspepsia may be caused by a variety of circumstances, but some frequent ones are:

1. Dietary Factors: Spicy and fatty meals, coffee, and alcohol may all increase dyspepsia symptoms. Individuals may find comfort by recognizing and avoiding foods that exacerbate their symptoms.

2. Poor lifestyle choices, such as overeating, eating too rapidly, and eating heavy meals before sleep,

may all lead to dyspepsia. Adopting better eating habits, such as eating smaller, more frequent meals and giving yourself enough time to digest before resting down may help relieve symptoms.

3. Underlying gastrointestinal diseases such as GERD, peptic ulcers, gastritis, and irritable bowel syndrome (IBS) may cause dyspepsia symptoms. Proper identification and treatment of these disorders are critical for adequate symptom relief and avoiding consequences.

4. Medications: Nonsteroidal anti-inflammatory medicines (NSAIDs), aspirin, and antibiotics may all irritate the stomach lining and cause dyspepsia. It is important to address possible pharmaceutical side effects with a healthcare professional and, if required, seek alternate treatment choices.

5. Psychological Factors: Stress, worry, and depression may all worsen dyspepsia symptoms by

impairing digestive function and raising sensitivity to pain. Stress-reduction approaches such as mindfulness, relaxation exercises, or therapy may assist control symptoms in those suffering from psychological discomfort.

Understanding the many causes of dyspepsia allows people to make proactive efforts to control their symptoms and improve their overall digestive health. Consulting with a healthcare expert for an accurate diagnosis and customized treatment suggestions is critical for treating underlying issues and providing long-term symptom alleviation.

CHAPTER 2

Digestive System Basics

Overview Of The Digestive System

Understanding dyspepsia requires an understanding of the digestive system, which is the mechanism by which our bodies process food. Consider it a well-orchestrated symphony of organs and systems, all working together to convert what we consume into nutrients that our bodies can absorb. The voyage begins in the mouth, where food is digested and combined with saliva, which includes enzymes that help break down carbs. It then goes down the throat into the stomach.

An essential part of the digestive process is the stomach. It functions similarly to a mixing bowl, blending food with digestive secretions rich in enzymes and acids.

This acidic atmosphere helps to break down meals into tiny pieces. Following the stomach, partly digested food enters the small intestine, where the majority of nutritional absorption occurs. The pancreas' digestive enzymes and the liver's bile help break down proteins, lipids, and carbs into molecules small enough to be absorbed into the circulation.

The small intestine is lined with millions of tiny finger-like extensions called villi, which increase surface area and aid in nutrition absorption. Any remaining indigestible material travels to the large intestine, where water and electrolytes are absorbed, and the waste is converted into stool. Finally, the waste is evacuated by the rectum and the anus.

How Digestion Works

Digestion is a complicated process that combines mechanical and chemical processes. Mechanical digestion starts in the mouth with chewing, which breaks down food into smaller pieces, making it simpler to swallow and exposing more surface area to digestive enzymes. Once in the stomach, the muscle walls flex and combine the food with digestive fluids, further breaking it down into a semi-liquid material known as chyme.

Chemical digestion is the process by which enzymes and acids break down food molecules into their smallest components. Proteins are degraded into amino acids, lipids into fatty acids and glycerol, and carbohydrates into simple sugars such as glucose. These smaller molecules are subsequently absorbed through the intestinal wall and into the circulation, where the body uses them for energy, growth, and repair.

Role Of Digestive Enzymes And Hormones

Digestive enzymes act as biochemical scissors in the digestive system. They accelerate the chemical processes that convert food into smaller molecules that can be absorbed. Each enzyme has a specialized function; for example, amylase breaks down carbohydrates, protease breaks down proteins, and lipase degrades lipids. The salivary glands, stomach, pancreas, and small intestine all manufacture these enzymes.

Hormones also play an important role in digestion, regulating the release of digestive fluids and the flow of food along the digestive system. For example, gastrin causes the stomach to create acid, while secretin and cholecystokinin cause the pancreas to release digestive enzymes and the gallbladder to secrete bile. These hormones ensure that digestion runs smoothly and effectively by coordinating the activity of many digestive organs to maximize nutrition absorption.

Understanding the fundamentals of the digestive system, how digestion works, and the functions of digestive enzymes and hormones lays the groundwork for understanding dyspepsia. Understanding how the digestive process should work normally allows us to better recognize and manage problems that occur when things go wrong, resulting in symptoms such as indigestion, bloating, and discomfort.

CHAPTER 3

Lifestyle Factors And Diet

Importance Of Diet In Digestive Health

Diet is essential for preserving digestive health, particularly when coping with dyspepsia. Dyspepsia, often known as indigestion, may be aggravated or relieved by certain meals. Understanding the effects of nutrition on digestive health is critical for successful dyspepsia management.

The foods we eat have a direct impact on how our digestive systems operate. Certain meals may irritate the stomach lining, causing symptoms including bloating, pain, and heartburn, which are frequent in dyspepsia. On the other side, a well-balanced, nutrient-dense diet may support good digestion and reduce the likelihood of feeling digestive pain.

Individuals who follow a stomach-friendly diet that supports regular digestion may greatly lessen the frequency and intensity of dyspeptic symptoms. This underlines the necessity of making educated food choices and developing good eating habits to improve overall digestive health.

Foods To Avoid And Foods To Embrace

When controlling dyspepsia with nutrition, it is important to be aware of the items that might exacerbate or relieve symptoms.

Foods To Avoid:

1. Spicy foods may irritate the stomach lining, increasing dyspepsia symptoms such as heartburn and acid reflux.

2. Fatty meals: High-fat meals, such as fried dishes and fatty meats, may cause stomach fullness and discomfort.

3. Acidic meals: Citrus fruits, tomatoes, and other acidic meals may raise stomach acid levels, causing indigestion.

4. Carbonated beverages may create bloating and gas, which can exacerbate dyspepsia symptoms.

5. Caffeine and alcohol may relax the lower esophageal sphincter, enabling stomach acid to enter the esophagus and produce pain.

Foods to embrace:

1. Fiber-rich meals including fruits, vegetables, and whole grains improve good digestion and help avoid constipation, which is a major cause of dyspepsia.

2. Lean Proteins: Choose lean protein sources including chicken, fish, tofu, and lentils, which are simpler to digest than fatty meat.

3. Probiotic-Rich Foods: Consuming probiotic-rich foods such as yogurt, kefir, and fermented vegetables may help to maintain a healthy balance of gut flora and aid digestion.

4. Low-Acid Options: To lessen the chance of discomfort, choose for low-acid alternatives to acidic meals such as non-citrus fruits and non-tomato sauces.

5. Herbal teas, such as chamomile, ginger, and peppermint, help relax the digestive tract and relieve dyspepsia.

Individuals may better manage dyspepsia and enhance their overall digestive health by being choosy about the meals they eat and choosing ones that are easy on the stomach.

Healthy Eating Habits For Managing Dyspepsia

In addition to being cautious of particular foods, maintaining good eating habits may help control dyspepsia.

1. Eat Smaller, More Regular Meals: **Rather than ingesting huge meals, which may place additional strain on the digestive system, choose smaller, more regular meals throughout the day. This method may assist to avoid stomach overload and reduce indigestion symptoms.**

2. Chew Food Thoroughly: **Properly chewing food before swallowing promotes digestion and minimizes the risk of bloating and discomfort.**

3. Avoid Eating Before Bed: **Give yourself enough time to digest by avoiding heavy meals and snacks close to sleep.**

Lying down quickly after eating might exacerbate dyspepsia symptoms, such as acid reflux.

4. **Stay Hydrated:** Drinking enough water throughout the day supports good digestion and prevents constipation, which is a major cause of indigestion.

5. **Manage Stress:** Dyspepsia symptoms might worsen while under stress. Incorporate stress-reduction strategies like deep breathing, meditation, or yoga into your routine to improve digestive health.

Individuals who practice these healthy eating habits may successfully control dyspepsia and improve overall digestive health. Making educated food choices and lifestyle changes may dramatically improve the quality of life for those suffering from stomach pain.

CHAPTER 4

Stress And Its Impact

Relationship Between Stress And Digestive Health

Understanding the complex link between stress and digestive health is critical for successful dyspepsia management. Stress has a tremendous influence on your body, especially your digestive system. When you are stressed, your body enters a state of heightened vigilance, which causes the production of chemicals such as cortisol and adrenaline. These hormones may alter the natural operation of your digestive organs, causing symptoms such as indigestion, bloating, and stomach pain.

Furthermore, stress might worsen pre-existing digestive problems including dyspepsia. Chronic stress may impair the immune system, increasing your susceptibility to gastrointestinal infections and inflammation. Furthermore, stress may affect the makeup of gut bacteria, which play an important role in digestion and health. Imbalances in gut microbiota have been related to a variety of digestive issues, including dyspepsia.

Recognizing how stress affects digestive health is the first step toward properly controlling dyspepsia. Addressing stress and practicing stress management practices may help you reduce symptoms and improve your overall well-being.

Stress Management Techniques

Stress management is vital for preserving digestive health and relieving dyspepsia symptoms. Fortunately, there are a variety of practices you may implement into your everyday routine to decrease stress and increase relaxation.

Deep breathing exercises are an efficient stress-management method. Deep breathing may assist in stimulating the body's relaxation response, which counteracts the effects of stress chemicals. To practice deep breathing, choose a quiet, comfortable area to sit or lie down. Close your eyes and take slow, deep breaths while concentrating on the feeling of air entering and exiting your body. Inhale deeply through your nose, filling your lungs with oxygen, then exhale slowly through your mouth, releasing tension with each breath.

Progressive muscle relaxation is another effective stress-management approach. This is systematically tensing and releasing various muscle groups in the body to induce both physical and mental calm. Begin by tensing the muscles in your feet, then gradually work your way up the body, tensing and releasing each group as you go. Pay attention to any areas of tension or pain, and let them go as you relax each muscle group.

In addition to these strategies, including mindfulness practices in your everyday routine may aid in stress reduction and digestive health. Mindfulness entails being in the present moment and paying attention to your thoughts, emotions, and body sensations without judgment. Meditation, yoga, and tai chi are all practices that may aid with dyspepsia symptoms by promoting awareness and relaxation.

By adopting stress management practices into your daily routine, you may decrease stress, relieve dyspepsia symptoms, and improve your overall health.

Mindfulness And Relaxation Exercises

Mindfulness and relaxation activities are effective strategies for stress management and digestive health. These techniques include becoming completely present in the moment while creating a feeling of tranquility and mindfulness.

Meditation is an excellent mindfulness practice. Meditation is concentrating your attention on a certain object, idea, or action, such as your breathing or a mantra. Meditation, by focusing your attention inward and letting go of distracting ideas, may help you relax and relieve tension. Even a few minutes of meditation every day may significantly improve your digestive health and general well-being.

Yoga is another effective way to promote calm. Yoga blends physical postures, breathing exercises, and meditation to help the body and mind achieve balance and harmony. Certain yoga positions may aid with dyspepsia symptoms by increasing digestion and relaxing the abdominal muscles. Gentle twists, forward folds, and backbends may aid enhance circulation to the digestive organs while also promoting relaxation.

Tai chi is another mindful activity that might improve intestinal health. Tai chi is a peaceful martial art that emphasizes calm, flowing motions and deep breathing. This exercise promotes relaxation, balance, and mental clarity, making it a great choice for stress management and digestive health.

Incorporating mindfulness and relaxation activities into your daily routine may help decrease stress, relieve dyspepsia symptoms, and improve your general well-being. Whether you prefer meditation, yoga, tai chi, or other mindfulness exercises, determining what works best for you is essential for boosting digestive health and well-being.

CHAPTER 5

Medications And Dyspepsia

Common Medications That Can Cause Dyspepsia

Dyspepsia, often known as indigestion, may be caused by a variety of circumstances, including certain drugs. Understanding which drugs may induce dyspepsia is critical for efficiently managing symptoms. Nonsteroidal anti-inflammatory medicines (NSAIDs) such as ibuprofen and aspirin, which are often used to treat pain, may irritate the stomach lining and cause indigestion. Furthermore, some antibiotics, such as erythromycin and tetracycline, might induce gastrointestinal problems in certain people. Bisphosphonates, which are used to treat osteoporosis, have also been linked to dyspepsia.

Furthermore, many cardiovascular medicines, such as calcium channel blockers and nitrates, may relax the muscles in the esophagus and stomach, possibly leading to acid reflux and dyspepsia symptoms. Furthermore, several mental drugs, such as antidepressants and antipsychotics, may impact the gastrointestinal tract, causing indigestion and pain. It is important to remember that individual reactions to drugs vary, and dyspepsia is not a common side effect. However, being aware of these possible triggers might assist people in better managing their symptoms.

How To Minimize Medication-Related Symptoms

If you have dyspepsia symptoms that you feel are caused by your drugs, you may use a variety of tactics to alleviate your discomfort. First and foremost, you must take your prescriptions exactly as directed by your healthcare professional.

Avoid changing the amount or frequency without first visiting your doctor, as this might worsen symptoms or lead to additional issues. Consider taking drugs with food or a full glass of water to help soothe the stomach and prevent inflammation.

Furthermore, if you're using NSAIDs for pain, talk to your doctor about alternatives like acetaminophen, which has fewer gastrointestinal adverse effects. If you are having dyspepsia symptoms as a result of antibiotics, your doctor may offer probiotics or antacids to help relieve the pain and restore balance to the gut microbiota. Furthermore, lifestyle changes such as avoiding hot or acidic meals, limiting alcohol use, and exercising stress-reduction strategies may help supplement medication management and enhance overall digestive health.

Consulting Your Doctor About Medication

If you have chronic dyspepsia symptoms or believe that your drugs are causing your discomfort, contact your doctor right away. Your doctor may do a comprehensive examination to establish the underlying cause of your symptoms and provide appropriate therapy recommendations. During your visit, be ready to offer extensive information about your medical history, including any drugs you are presently taking, as well as precise details about your symptoms and their intensity.

Your doctor may suggest changing your drug regimen, suggesting alternate therapies, or sending you to a gastroenterologist for additional testing. Open and honest communication with your healthcare practitioner is critical to getting the most effective treatment suited to your specific requirements. Furthermore, follow-up sessions may be required to assess your progress and make any necessary changes to your treatment strategy. Working together with your doctor allows you to properly control dyspepsia symptoms while also improving your overall quality of life.

CHAPTER 6

Natural Remedies And Supplements

Herbal Remedies For Dyspepsia

When it comes to treating dyspepsia, herbal treatments provide a natural and generally mild way to relieve stomach distress. Ginger is a popular herb with digestive effects. Ginger includes anti-inflammatory chemicals such as gingerol and school, which may help relieve bloating and nausea. Making a cup of ginger tea or even chewing on a piece of fresh ginger might provide comfort.

Peppermint is another popular herb for relieving dyspepsia. Peppermint includes menthol, which relaxes the muscles of the digestive system and may help with cramping and bloating. Drinking peppermint tea or taking peppermint oil capsules before meals may help to alleviate dyspeptic symptoms.

Chamomile is another plant that has been shown to have calming effects on the mind and stomach. Chamomile tea is often used to ease stress and anxiety, which might aggravate digestive problems. Its anti-inflammatory effects may also aid in soothe an upset stomach and relieve flatulence.

In addition to these regularly used herbs, fennel, licorice root, and lemon balm may help relieve dyspepsia symptoms. However, before adding any herbal therapies into your daily routine, you should contact a healthcare expert, particularly if you are pregnant, nursing, or using drugs that may interfere with these herbs.

Probiotics And Digestive Health

Probiotics, sometimes known as "good" bacteria, are essential for gastrointestinal health. These living microbes are present in fermented foods such as yogurt, kefir, sauerkraut, and kimchi, as well as in supplements. Probiotics assist in restoring the balance of bacteria in the gut, which may be disturbed by stress, disease, or a bad diet.

According to research, probiotics may aid with dyspepsia symptoms by lowering inflammation in the digestive system and facilitating regular bowel movements. They may also improve nutrition absorption and gastrointestinal function.

When selecting a probiotic supplement, seek one that has a range of bacterial strains, such as Lactobacillus and Bifidobacterium species. Begin with a modest dosage and increase gradually as tolerated. Probiotics must also be consumed regularly to retain their digestive benefits.

Probiotics may be added to your diet in the form of yogurt with live cultures or a regular probiotic pill. However, if you have underlying health concerns or are immunocompromised, you should visit a healthcare expert before beginning any new supplements.

Integrating Supplements Safely

While natural therapies and supplements might help with dyspepsia symptoms, it's important to include them carefully in your regimen. Here are some suggestions for doing so:

1. Consult with a healthcare professional: Before beginning any new supplement regimen, speak with your doctor or another experienced healthcare practitioner.

They may provide individualized advice based on your medical history and specific requirements.

2. **Investigate possible interactions:** Some supplements may interfere with drugs or worsen existing health concerns. Before adding a new supplement to your regimen, be sure you've researched any possible interactions.

3. When taking a new supplement, begin with a low dosage and gradually increase as tolerated. This reduces the chance of negative effects and allows you to monitor how your body reacts.

4. **Monitor for adverse effects:** Keep an eye out for any changes or side effects that occur after beginning a new supplement. If you have any side effects, stop using it and see a doctor.

5. **Give it time:** Natural therapies and supplements may need some time to take action. Be patient and

persistent with your program, and allow your body time to adapt.

By following these instructions and consulting with a healthcare practitioner, you may safely include natural therapies and supplements into your daily routine to improve digestive health and control dyspepsia symptoms.

CHAPTER 7

Diagnosing Dyspepsia

Medical Tests For Identifying Dyspepsia

When it comes to diagnosing dyspepsia, healthcare experts utilize several medical tests to determine the origin of the symptoms. These tests are critical in determining an accurate diagnosis and a successful treatment strategy. Let's look at some of the most popular medical tests used to diagnose dyspepsia.

Upper Endoscopy: This technique includes putting a thin, flexible tube with a camera (endoscope) down the neck to view the esophagus, stomach, and upper section of the small intestine. It enables the healthcare professional to visually examine the lining of these organs for abnormalities such as inflammation, ulcers, or tumors.

Upper GI Series: Also known as a barium swallow, this test requires ingesting a chalky liquid containing barium while X-rays are collected. Barium covers the linings of the esophagus, stomach, and small intestine, making them visible on X-ray imaging. This aids in discovering structural problems or obstructions that might be producing dyspepsia symptoms.

Blood testing may help uncover underlying diseases like H. pylori infection, anemia, or pancreatitis that might be causing dyspepsia symptoms. These tests may include a complete blood count (CBC), pancreatic enzyme levels, and particular antibodies.

Stool Tests: Stool tests are often conducted to detect the presence of H. pylori bacteria or indications of gastrointestinal bleeding, which might indicate certain digestive diseases that cause dyspepsia.

Breath Tests: Breath tests identify the presence of H. pylori bacteria by testing breath samples taken before and after consuming a specialized solution. This noninvasive test may provide important information regarding the existence of H. pylori infection is a frequent cause of dyspepsia.

Consulting With Healthcare Professionals

When suffering dyspepsia symptoms, it is important to seek medical advice to have an accurate diagnosis and treatment. Here's a guide for consulting with healthcare specialists about dyspepsia.

Main Care Physician: Make an appointment with your main care physician. They will thoroughly assess your symptoms, and medical history, and do a physical examination. Based on their findings, they may suggest more diagnostic testing or send you to a specialist.

If your primary care physician feels that your dyspepsia symptoms are caused by an underlying gastrointestinal illness, he or she may recommend you to a gastroenterologist. These professionals are trained to diagnose and treat digestive-related diseases. A gastroenterologist may order further tests, such as an endoscopy or imaging scans, to determine the origin of your symptoms further.

Nutritionist or Dietitian: In certain circumstances, dietary considerations might exacerbate dyspepsia symptoms. Consulting with a nutritionist or dietitian may help you identify trigger foods and make dietary changes to ease symptoms. They may provide unique dietary suggestions based on your particular requirements and lifestyle.

Psychologist or Psychiatrist: Emotional stress and psychological issues might worsen dyspepsia symptoms in certain people. If stress or anxiety are considered to be contributing factors, seeing a psychologist or psychiatrist may assist address these concerns via treatment, relaxation methods, or medication, as needed.

Understanding Diagnostic Procedures

Navigating diagnostic tests for dyspepsia may be intimidating, but knowing the goal and method of each test can help reduce anxiety and improve communication with healthcare specialists. Here's an overview of typical diagnostic methods used to diagnose dyspepsia.

Process Explanation: Before any diagnostic test, your healthcare professional will explain the objective of the process, what to anticipate during the test, and any necessary preparations. Don't be afraid to ask inquiries if anything is confusing.

Informed Consent: Informed consent is a vital component of the diagnostic procedure. Before consenting to the operation, it is necessary to understand its dangers, advantages, and alternatives. Your healthcare professional will make sure you are completely informed and comfortable before beginning with the test.

Patient Preparation: Depending on the kind of diagnostic test, you may be required to follow certain preparation guidelines. This may involve fasting for a certain length of time before the test, quitting specific medicines, or abstaining from foods or beverages that might affect the findings.

During the Procedure: Healthcare personnel will make sure you're comfortable and safe. They will offer directions and supervision during the procedure, and you may be sedated or anesthetized for some procedures, such as an endoscope.

Post-Procedure Care: After the test, your healthcare professional will discuss the results with you and any further actions or treatments that may be required based on them. They will also provide you with post-procedure instructions and warn you about any possible adverse effects.

Understanding the diagnostic processes for dyspepsia might help you take an active part in your healthcare journey. Working cooperatively with your healthcare team and remaining educated will allow you to confidently navigate the diagnostic process and concentrate on symptom alleviation.

CHAPTER 8

Treatment Options

Lifestyle Changes For Managing Dyspepsia

When it comes to controlling dyspepsia, lifestyle adjustments may help alleviate symptoms and improve overall health. These modifications are often the first line of defense and may be quite successful if performed regularly.

Dietary Adjustments: Modifying your food is one of the most important lifestyle modifications. Certain meals and drinks may cause or worsen dyspeptic symptoms. Spicy, fatty, and acidic meals, as well as coffee and alcohol, are prominent triggers. Instead, aim for a well-balanced diet high in fruits, vegetables, lean meats, and healthy grains. Eating smaller, more frequent meals might also assist in alleviating pain.

Meal Timing and Portions: Keep track of when and how much you consume. Eating too rapidly or too close to sleep might stress your digestive system, causing pain. Try to eat at regular intervals and avoid large meals late at night.

Stress Management: Because stress is so directly tied to digestive health, learning how to control it may be helpful. Incorporate relaxation practices like deep breathing, meditation, yoga, or mild movement into your regular schedule. Participating in hobbies or activities you like may also assist in relieving stress.

Weight Management: Keeping a healthy weight is critical for general health, including digestion. Excess weight may put a strain on the stomach, worsening dyspepsia symptoms. To acquire and maintain a healthy weight, follow a well-balanced diet and get frequent exercise.

Smoking cessation: Smoking has been demonstrated to raise the likelihood of dyspeptic symptoms and may also impair the efficacy of certain therapies. Quitting smoking may significantly enhance intestinal health and general well-being.

Avoiding Cause Substances: Determine which substances cause or aggravate your symptoms and avoid them wherever feasible. Some medicines, such as nonsteroidal anti-inflammatory drugs (NSAIDs) or aspirin, might irritate the stomach lining.

water: Proper digestion requires enough water, which may help ease dyspepsia symptoms. Aim to drink lots of water throughout the day and avoid carbonated drinks, which may cause gas and bloating.

Implementing these lifestyle adjustments allows you to actively manage your dyspepsia and improve your quality of life.

Medical Treatments And Procedures

In addition to lifestyle adjustments, medical treatments, and procedures may be required to properly manage dyspepsia, particularly if symptoms are severe or continue after lifestyle improvements.

Antacids: Over-the-counter antacids may give immediate relief from symptoms by neutralizing stomach acid. These drugs are often used as required to treat occasional bouts of indigestion or heartburn.

Proton Pump Inhibitors (PPIs): PPIs are drugs that lower stomach acid production and are frequently used to treat gastroesophageal reflux disease (GERD) and peptic ulcers.

They may also help with dyspepsia symptoms, especially if acid reflux is a significant problem.

Histamine-2 Receptor Antagonists (H2RAs) are another kind of medicine that lowers stomach acid production. They may be used as a substitute for PPIs or in conjunction with other drugs to treat symptoms.

Prokinetic Agents: These drugs increase gastric emptying and gastrointestinal motility, which may benefit certain dyspepsia patients, especially those who have delayed gastric emptying.

Antibiotics: If dyspepsia is caused by an infection with Helicobacter pylori bacteria, antibiotics may be recommended to treat the infection and relieve symptoms.

Endoscopic Procedures: In certain circumstances, endoscopy may be indicated to examine the esophagus, stomach, and duodenum for abnormalities or underlying disorders that may be causing dyspepsia. During an endoscopy, a thin, flexible tube with a camera attached (endoscope) is passed via the mouth and into the digestive system, enabling the doctor to visually evaluate the lining of the digestive organs and collect tissue samples as needed.

Surgery: In rare situations, if dyspepsia is caused by structural abnormalities or consequences such as gastric outlet blockage, surgery may be required to address the underlying problem.

Developing A Personalized Treatment Plan

Dyspepsia care frequently requires an individualized strategy based on the patient's symptoms, underlying reasons, and medical history. A thorough treatment approach may include a variety of lifestyle changes, medicines, and perhaps procedural procedures.

The first stage in creating a tailored treatment plan is a complete medical examination by a healthcare practitioner. This may involve a thorough medical history, a physical examination, and maybe diagnostic procedures such as blood tests, imaging investigations, or endoscopy.

Collaborative Decision-Making: Treatment choices should be made in partnership with the patient and their healthcare practitioner. They may review the various treatment choices, consider the advantages and risks, and create a strategy that is tailored to the patient's preferences and objectives.

Regular Follow-Up: Dyspepsia is a chronic illness for many people, and continuing treatment may be required to control symptoms and avoid consequences.

Regular follow-up meetings with a healthcare professional are critical for tracking improvement, adjusting therapy as required, and addressing any new or persistent problems.

Patient Education: Providing patients with information about their disease and treatment choices is critical for effective dyspepsia management. Patients should be informed of the necessity of making lifestyle changes, adhering to drug regimens, and recognizing warning signals that may suggest the need for medical care.

Multidisciplinary Approach: In certain circumstances, controlling dyspepsia may need the collaboration of many healthcare specialists, including gastroenterologists, nutritionists, psychologists, and surgeons. A multidisciplinary approach may provide complete treatment while addressing all elements of the patient's health and well-being.

CHAPTER 9

Preventing Dyspepsia

Strategies For Preventing Recurrence

Preventing dyspepsia recurrence requires a multimodal strategy that tackles both lifestyle and underlying medical issues. One of the most important techniques is food change. Certain meals and drinks, including spicy foods, citrus fruits, caffeine, and alcohol, may cause dyspeptic symptoms in sensitive people. Avoiding these triggers and eating a bland diet high in fruits, vegetables, healthy grains, and lean meats will help to reduce symptom flare-ups.

Stress management is also an important part of prevention. Stress may increase digestive difficulties and worsen dyspepsia symptoms. Incorporating stress-reduction practices like mindfulness meditation, deep breathing exercises, yoga, or regular physical activity into your daily routine will help reduce stress and its effects on your digestive system.

Maintaining a healthy weight is also crucial for avoiding dyspepsia. Excess weight may put a strain on the stomach and raise the chance of acid reflux, which can cause or exacerbate dyspeptic symptoms. A balanced diet and regular exercise will help you reach and maintain a healthy weight, lowering your chance of dyspepsia recurrence.

In addition to dietary and lifestyle changes, it is critical to address any underlying medical issues that may contribute to dyspepsia. This may include treating disorders like gastroesophageal reflux disease (GERD), peptic ulcers, or Helicobacter pylori infection using medication, lifestyle modifications, or other treatments suggested by your healthcare physician.

Regular follow-up with your healthcare practitioner is essential for evaluating your symptoms and changing your treatment plan as necessary. Your doctor may prescribe regular testing, such as an endoscopy or imaging test, to monitor the health of your digestive system and detect any possible issues or changes that may need action.

By applying these techniques and collaborating closely with your healthcare team, you may lower the risk of dyspepsia recurrence while also improving your digestive health and general well-being.

Long-Term Management Techniques

Dyspepsia requires long-term therapy that includes continual monitoring, lifestyle changes, and adherence to treatment recommendations to reduce symptoms and avoid complications. Long-term treatment includes recognizing and avoiding trigger foods and drinks that might aggravate dyspeptic symptoms. Keeping a food diary might help you monitor your diet and find correlations between certain meals and symptom flare-ups.

In addition to dietary changes, a healthy lifestyle is essential for long-term dyspepsia treatment. This includes regular exercise, stress management strategies, getting enough sleep, and avoiding tobacco and excessive alcohol intake. These lifestyle variables may have an impact on digestive health and aid in avoiding dyspepsia recurrence.

Medication management is another important aspect of long-term treatment for those who have chronic or recurrent dyspepsia. Depending on the underlying cause of dyspepsia, your doctor may recommend proton pump inhibitors (PPIs), H2 receptor antagonists, antacids, prokinetics, or antibiotics for Helicobacter pylori infection. It is important to take your medicines exactly as recommended and to mention any changes in symptoms or adverse effects to your healthcare practitioner.

Regular follow-up consultations with your healthcare practitioner are critical for monitoring your symptoms, assessing therapy efficacy, and changing your management strategy as required. Your doctor may prescribe regular testing, such as an endoscopy or imaging test, to check the health of your digestive system and detect any changes or abnormalities that may need action.

In certain circumstances, lifestyle changes and medication management may not be sufficient to bring relief, necessitating further measures. These therapies may involve surgical procedures, such as fundoplication for GERD or pyloroplasty for gastroparesis, to address underlying anatomical or functional defects that cause dyspepsia symptoms.

Overall, long-term dyspepsia care requires a comprehensive strategy that includes lifestyle changes, medication management, and frequent monitoring to reduce symptoms, avoid complications, and improve quality of life.

Incorporating Healthy Habits Into Daily Life

Incorporating good behaviors into your daily routine is critical for avoiding dyspepsia and improving overall digestive health. One of the most essential habits is to eat a well-balanced diet rich in fruits, vegetables, whole grains, and lean meats while avoiding foods and drinks that aggravate dyspeptic symptoms. Eating modest, frequent meals throughout the day and avoiding big meals or heavy snacks before sleep might also assist in alleviating pain and aid digestion.

Staying hydrated is an important element of digestive health. Drinking enough water throughout the day may help avoid constipation and encourage regular bowel movements, lowering the risk of dyspepsia and other gastrointestinal problems. Limiting your consumption of carbonated beverages, caffeinated drinks, and alcohol may also help avoid dehydration and stomach issues.

Regular physical exercise is crucial for good health and digestive function. Exercise may accelerate digestion, enhance gastrointestinal motility, and decrease stress, all of which can assist in maintaining a healthy digestive tract. Aim for at least 30 minutes of moderate-intensity activity on most days of the week, such as brisk walking, cycling, swimming, or aerobic exercise courses.

In addition to nutrition and exercise, stress management is essential for avoiding dyspepsia and improving digestive health. Stress may interfere with regular digestive processes, exacerbating dyspepsia symptoms. Incorporating stress-reduction practices like mindfulness meditation, deep breathing exercises, yoga, or progressive muscle relaxation into your daily routine may help relieve stress and promote relaxation, which is good for your digestive system.

Adequate sleep is also beneficial to digestive health. Poor or insufficient sleep may disturb hormone levels, metabolism, and immune function, affecting digestive health and contributing to dyspeptic symptoms. Aim for seven to nine hours of quality sleep every night by following excellent sleep hygiene behaviors such as sticking to a regular sleep schedule, developing a calming bedtime ritual, and establishing a pleasant sleep environment.

CHAPTER 10

Living Well With Dyspepsia
Coping Strategies For Daily Life

Living with dyspepsia may be difficult daily, but there are coping methods available to assist in controlling symptoms and enhance quality of life. One useful method is to identify and avoid meals and drinks that worsen symptoms. Keeping a food journal might help identify particular triggers. Additionally, mindful eating, which entails eating slowly and carefully, might help digestion and alleviate pain.

Another coping approach is to make lifestyle changes that improve gut health. This involves maintaining a healthy weight by regular exercise and consuming a well-balanced diet high in fiber, fruits, and vegetables. Avoiding heavy meals, particularly before sleep, may help relieve symptoms by lowering stomach pressure and minimizing acid reflux.

Incorporating stress-reduction practices into everyday life might also help manage dyspepsia symptoms. Stress has been related to digestive problems, so finding techniques to relax and unwind, such as yoga, meditation, or deep breathing exercises, might help ease symptoms. Creating a relaxing evening routine and getting enough sleep might help with intestinal health.

It is critical to collaborate closely with healthcare specialists to create a specific treatment strategy for dyspepsia symptoms. This might include drugs to lower stomach acid, relieve discomfort, or address underlying diseases like H. Helicobacter pylori infection. Regular check-ups with a healthcare practitioner may assist in monitoring symptoms and adjusting therapy as necessary.

Support Networks And Resources

Living with dyspepsia may be isolated, but there are support networks and services available to assist people deal with their disease. Support groups, whether in person or online, may provide a feeling of community and solidarity among others experiencing similar issues. Sharing your experiences, insights, and coping tactics with others may be both powerful and affirming.

In addition to peer support, healthcare professionals play an important role in offering assistance and resources for dyspepsia treatment. Gastroenterologists, nutritionists, and mental health specialists may provide specialized guidance based on individual requirements. They may also give educational materials, seminars, and other tools to help people understand and manage dyspepsia.

Individuals with dyspepsia must advocate for themselves and seek necessary help. This might include asking questions during medical visits, requesting referrals to experts, or contacting support groups for more help. Individuals who actively engage with their healthcare team and support network may feel more empowered to properly manage their illness.

Thriving Despite Digestive Challenges

Living with dyspepsia may be difficult, but it is possible to flourish and enjoy life despite digestive problems. Maintaining a good perspective and concentrating on what one can control is essential for prospering. This involves developing good living choices, requesting help when necessary, and being proactive in controlling symptoms.

Setting realistic objectives and expectations might help you thrive with dyspepsia. Recognizing that there will be good and bad days, as well as being compassionate with oneself during flare-ups, might help to avoid emotions of anger or disappointment. Celebrating even tiny successes and achievements may increase morale and motivation.

Finding delight in activities that provide pleasure and satisfaction may improve general well-being. Prioritizing self-care and pleasure, whether by spending time with loved ones, following hobbies and interests, or indulging in creative activities, may help to alleviate the difficulties of living with dyspepsia. Creating a support network of understanding friends and family members may provide encouragement and aid during trying times.

Finally, surviving despite digestive issues requires a mix of self-care, support, and tenacity. Individuals with dyspepsia may have satisfying and meaningful lives by taking proactive actions to control their symptoms, getting help from healthcare experts and peers, and having a positive attitude.

CONCLUSION

To summarize, dyspepsia is a multidimensional ailment marked by discomfort or pain in the upper abdomen, which is often accompanied by symptoms such as bloating, nausea, and heartburn. Its causes are many, including nutrition, lifestyle, psychological stress, and underlying medical problems such as GERD, peptic ulcer disease, or gastritis.

Dyspepsia is diagnosed with a detailed medical history, physical examination, and, in some cases, further testing like as endoscopy, imaging scans, or laboratory tests to rule out other possible causes. Treatment techniques attempt to ease symptoms and treat underlying causes, which may include lifestyle changes, dietary changes, medication, or, in extreme situations, surgical intervention.

Despite its prevalence and effect on quality of life, dyspepsia remains difficult to control because of its heterogeneity and variable responsiveness to therapy. Additionally, the comorbidity with other gastrointestinal illnesses complicates diagnosis and therapy even more.

Moving ahead, continuing study into the pathophysiology of dyspepsia, as well as the development of more focused therapeutics, are critical for improving patient outcomes and quality of life. Furthermore, teaching patients about lifestyle changes and stress management approaches might help them better control their symptoms and lessen the need for medication treatments.

In clinical practice, a holistic approach that takes into account the biopsychosocial components of dyspepsia is essential for delivering complete therapy and meeting patients' different requirements. Collaboration among healthcare practitioners, researchers, and patients is critical for improving our knowledge and treatment of dyspepsia, eventually leading to better results and a higher quality of life for those suffering from this prevalent gastrointestinal condition.

THE END

www.ingramcontent.com/pod-product-compliance
Lightning Source LLC
Chambersburg PA
CBHW070314230526
45470CB00002B/879